How To Get Rid Of Heartburn Acid Reflux

337 Great Tips For Acid Reflux and Heartburn Relief

ADAM COLTON

Published by BizMove
www.bizmove.com

ISBN: 1978320272
ISBN- 978-1978320277

Table of Contents

1. Acid Reflux Fact Sheet

Gastroesophageal reflux (GER) happens when your stomach contents come back up into your esophagus.

Stomach acid that touches the lining of your esophagus can cause heartburn, also called acid indigestion.

Does GER have another name?

Doctors also refer to GER as

- acid indigestion
- acid reflux
- acid regurgitation
- heartburn
- reflux

How common is GER?

Having GER once in a while is common.

What is GERD?

Gastroesophageal reflux disease (GERD) is a more serious and long-lasting form of GER.

What is the difference between **GER** and **GERD?**

GER that occurs more than twice a week for a few weeks could be GERD. GERD can lead to more serious health problems over time. If you think you have GERD, you should see your doctor.

How common is **GERD?**

GERD affects about 20 percent of the U.S. population.[1]

Who is more likely to have **GERD?**

Anyone can develop GERD, some for unknown reasons. You are more likely to have GERD if you are

- overweight or obese
- a pregnant woman
- taking certain medicines
- a smoker or regularly exposed to secondhand smoke

What are the complications of **GERD?**

Without treatment, GERD can sometimes cause serious complications over time, such as

Esophagitis

Esophagitis is inflammation in the esophagus. Adults who have chronic esophagitis over many years are more likely to develop precancerous changes in the esophagus.

Esophageal stricture

An esophageal stricture happens when your esophagus becomes too narrow. Esophageal strictures can lead to problems with swallowing.

Respiratory problems

With GERD you might breathe stomach acid into your lungs. The stomach acid can then irritate your throat and lungs, causing respiratory problems, such as

- asthma —a long-lasting disease in your lungs that makes you extra sensitive to things that you're allergic to
- chest congestion, or extra fluid in your lungs
- a dry, long-lasting cough or a sore throat
- hoarseness—the partial loss of your voice
- laryngitis—the swelling of your voice box that can lead to a short-term loss of your voice
- pneumonia—an infection in one or both of your lungs—that keeps coming back

- wheezing—a high-pitched whistling sound when you breathe

Barrett's esophagus

GERD can sometimes cause Barrett's esophagus. A small number of people with Barrett's esophagus develop a rare yet often deadly type of cancer of the esophagus.

If you have GERD, talk with your doctor about how to prevent or treat long-term problems.

What are the symptoms of GER and GERD?

If you have gastroesophageal reflux (GER), you may taste food or stomach acid in the back of your mouth.

The most common symptom of gastroesophageal reflux disease (GERD) is regular heartburn, a painful, burning feeling in the middle of your chest, behind your breastbone, and in the middle of your abdomen. Not all adults with GERD have heartburn.

Other common GERD symptoms include

- bad breath
- nausea

- pain in your chest or the upper part of your abdomen
- problems swallowing or painful swallowing
- respiratory problems
- vomiting
- the wearing away of your teeth

Some symptoms of GERD come from its complications, including those that affect your lungs.

What causes GER and GERD?

GER and GERD happen when your lower esophageal sphincter becomes weak or relaxes when it shouldn't, causing stomach contents to rise up into the esophagus. The lower esophageal sphincter becomes weak or relaxes due to certain things, such as

- increased pressure on your abdomen from being overweight, obese, or pregnant
- certain medicines, including
    - those that doctors use to treat asthma —a long-lasting disease in your lungs that makes you extra sensitive to things that you're allergic to
    - calcium channel blockers—medicines that treat high blood pressure

- o antihistamines—medicines that treat allergy symptoms
  - o painkillers
  - o sedatives—medicines that help put you to sleep
  - o antidepressants —medicines that treat depression
- smoking, or inhaling secondhand smoke

A hiatal hernia can also cause GERD. Hiatal hernia is a condition in which the opening in your diaphragm lets the upper part of the stomach move up into your chest, which lowers the pressure in the esophageal sphincter.

When should I seek a doctor's help?

You should see a doctor if you have persistent GER symptoms that do not get better with over-the-counter medications or change in your diet.

Call a doctor right away if you

- vomit large amounts
- have regular projectile, or forceful, vomiting
- vomit fluid that is
  - o green or yellow
  - o looks like coffee grounds
  - o contains blood
- have problems breathing after vomiting
- have pain in the mouth or throat when you eat

- have problems swallowing or painful swallowing

How do doctors diagnose GER?

In most cases, your doctor diagnoses gastroesophageal reflux (GER) by reviewing your symptoms and medical history. If your symptoms don't improve with lifestyle changes and medications, you may need testing.

How do doctors diagnose GERD?

If your GER symptoms don't improve, if they come back frequently, or if you have trouble swallowing, your doctor may recommend testing you for gastroesophageal reflux disease (GERD).

Your doctor may refer you to a gastroenterologist to diagnose and treat GERD.

What tests do doctors use to diagnose GERD?

Several tests can help a doctor diagnose GERD. Your doctor may order more than one test to make a diagnosis.

Upper gastrointestinal (GI) endoscopy and biopsy

In an upper GI endoscopy, a gastroenterologist, surgeon, or other trained health care professional uses an endoscope to see inside your upper GI tract. This procedure takes place at a hospital or an outpatient center.

An intravenous (IV) needle will be placed in your arm to provide a sedative. Sedatives help you stay relaxed and comfortable during the procedure. In some cases, the procedure can be performed without sedation. You will be given a liquid anesthetic to gargle or spray anesthetic on the back of your throat. The doctor carefully feeds the endoscope down your esophagus and into your stomach and duodenum. A small camera mounted on the endoscope sends a video image to a monitor, allowing close examination of the lining of your upper GI tract. The endoscope pumps air into your stomach and duodenum, making them easier to see.

The doctor may perform a biopsy with the endoscope by taking a small piece of tissue from the lining of your esophagus. You won't feel the biopsy. A pathologist examines the tissue in a lab.

In most cases, the procedure only diagnoses GERD if you have moderate to severe symptoms.

Read more about upper GI endoscopy.

Upper GI series

An upper GI series looks at the shape of your upper GI tract.

An x-ray technician performs this procedure at a hospital or an outpatient center. A radiologist reads and reports on the x-ray images. You don't need anesthesia. A health care professional will tell you how to prepare for the procedure, including when to stop eating and drinking.

During the procedure, you will stand or sit in front of an x-ray machine and drink barium to coat the inner lining of your upper GI tract. The x-ray technician takes several x-rays as the barium moves through your GI tract. The upper GI series can't show GERD in your esophagus; rather, the barium shows up on the x-ray and can find problems related to GERD, such as

- hiatal hernias
- esophageal strictures
- ulcers

You may have bloating and nausea for a short time after the procedure. For several days afterward, you may have white or light-colored stools from the barium. A health care professional will give you instructions about eating, drinking, and taking your medicines after the procedure.

Esophageal pH and impedance monitoring

The most accurate procedure to detect acid reflux is esophageal pH and impedance monitoring. Esophageal pH and impedance monitoring measures the amount of acid in your esophagus while you do normal things, such as eating and sleeping.

A gastroenterologist performs this procedure at a hospital or an outpatient center as a part of an upper GI endoscopy. Most often, you can stay awake during the procedure.

A gastroenterologist will pass a thin tube through your nose or mouth into your stomach. The gastroenterologist will then pull the tube back into your esophagus and tape it to your cheek. The end of the tube in your esophagus measures when and how much acid comes up your esophagus. The other end of the tube attaches to a monitor outside your body that records the measurements.

You will wear a monitor for the next 24 hours. You will return to the hospital or outpatient center to have the tube removed.

This procedure is most useful to your doctor if you keep a diary of when, what, and how much food you eat and your GERD symptoms are after you eat. The gastroenterologist can see how your symptoms, certain foods, and certain times of day relate to one another. The procedure can also help show whether acid reflux triggers any respiratory symptoms.

Bravo wireless esophageal pH monitoring

Bravo wireless esophageal pH monitoring also measures and records the pH in your esophagus to determine if you have GERD. A doctor temporarily attaches a small capsule to the wall of your esophagus during an upper endoscopy. The capsule measures pH levels in the esophagus and transmits information to a receiver. The receiver is about the size of a pager, which you wear on your belt or waistband.

You will follow your usual daily routine during monitoring, which usually lasts 48 hours. The receiver has several buttons on it that you will press to record symptoms of GERD such as heartburn. The nurse will tell you what symptoms to record. You will be asked to maintain a diary to record certain events such as when you start and stop eating and drinking, when you lie down, and when you get back up.

To prepare for the test talk to your doctor about medicines you are taking. He or she will tell you whether you can eat or drink before the procedure. After about seven to ten days the capsule will fall off the esophageal lining and pass through your digestive tract.

Esophageal manometry

Esophageal manometry measures muscle contractions in your esophagus. A gastroenterologist may order this procedure if you're thinking about anti-reflux surgery.

The gastroenterologist can perform this procedure during an office visit. A health care professional will spray a liquid anesthetic on the back of your throat or ask you to gargle a liquid anesthetic.

The gastroenterologist passes a soft, thin tube through your nose and into your stomach. You swallow as the gastroenterologist pulls the tube slowly back into your esophagus. A computer measures and records the pressure of muscle contractions in different parts of your esophagus.

The procedure can show if your symptoms are due to a weak sphincter muscle. A doctor can also use the procedure to diagnose other esophagus problems that might have symptoms similar to heartburn. A health care professional will give you instructions about eating, drinking, and taking your medicines after the procedure.

Treatment for **GER & GERD**

How do you control **GER** and **GERD?**

You may be able to control gastroesophageal reflux (GER) and gastroesophageal reflux disease (GERD) by

- not eating or drinking items that may cause GER, such as greasy or spicy foods and alcoholic drinks
- not overeating
- not eating 2 to 3 hours before bedtime
- losing weight if you're overweight or obese
- quitting smoking and avoiding secondhand smoke
- taking over-the-counter medicines, such as Maalox , or Rolaids

How do doctors treat **GERD?**

Depending on the severity of your symptoms, your doctor may recommend lifestyle changes, medicines, surgery, or a combination.

Lifestyle changes

Making lifestyle changes can reduce your GER and GERD symptoms. You should

- lose weight, if needed.
- wear loose-fitting clothing around your abdomen. Tight clothing can squeeze your stomach area and push acid up into your esophagus.
- stay upright for 3 hours after meals. Avoid reclining and slouching when sitting.
- sleep on a slight angle. Raise the head of your bed 6 to 8 inches by safely putting blocks under the bedposts. Just using extra pillows will not help.
- quit smoking and avoid secondhand smoke.

Over-the-counter and prescription medicines

You can buy many GERD medicines without a prescription. However, if you have symptoms that will not go away, you should see your doctor.

All GERD medicines work in different ways. You may need a combination of GERD medicines to control your symptoms.

Antacids. Doctors often first recommend antacids to relieve heartburn and other mild GER and

GERD symptoms. Antacids include over-the-counter medicines such as

- Maalox
- Mylanta
- Riopan
- Rolaids

Antacids can have side effects, including diarrhea and constipation.

H2 blockers. H2 blockers decrease acid production. They provide short-term or on-demand relief for many people with GER and GERD symptoms. They can also help heal the esophagus, although not as well as other medicines. You can buy H2 blockers over-the-counter or your doctor can prescribe one. Types of H2 blockers include

- cimetidine (Tagamet HB)
- famotidine (Pepcid AC)
- nizatidine (Axid AR)
- ranitidine (Zantac 75)

If you get heartburn after eating, your doctor may recommend that you take an antacid and an H2 blocker. The antacid neutralizes stomach acid, and the H2 blocker stops your stomach from creating acid. By the time the antacid stops working, the H2 blocker has stopped the acid.

Proton pump inhibitors (PPIs). PPIs lower the amount of acid your stomach makes. PPIs are better at treating GERD symptoms than H2 blockers.[2] They can heal the esophageal lining in most people with GERD. Doctors often prescribe PPIs for long-term GERD treatment.

However, studies show that people who take PPIs for a long time or in high doses are more likely to have hip, wrist, and spinal fractures. You need to take these medicines on an empty stomach so that your stomach acid can make them work.

Several types of PPIs are available by a doctor's prescription, including

- esomeprazole (Nexium)
- lansoprazole (Prevacid)
- omeprazole (Prilosec, Zegerid)
- pantoprazole (Protonix)
- rabeprazole (AcipHex)

Talk with your doctor about taking lower-strength omeprazole or lansoprazole, sold over the counter.

Prokinetics. Prokinetics help your stomach empty faster. Prescription prokinetics include

- bethanechol (Urecholine)
- metoclopramide (Reglan)

Both of these medicines have side effects, including

- nausea
- diarrhea
- fatigue, or feeling tired
- depression
- anxiety
- delayed or abnormal physical movement

Prokinetics can cause problems if you mix them with other medicines, so tell your doctor about all the medicines you're taking.

Antibiotics. Antibiotics, including erythromycin , can help your stomach empty faster. Erythromycin has fewer side effects than prokinetics; however, it can cause diarrhea.

Surgery

Your doctor may recommend surgery if your GERD symptoms don't improve with lifestyle changes or medicines. You're more likely to develop complications from surgery than from medicines.

Fundoplication is the most common surgery for GERD. In most cases, it leads to long-term reflux control.

A surgeon performs fundoplication using a laparoscope, a thin tube with a tiny video camera.

During the operation, a surgeon sews the top of your stomach around your esophagus to add pressure to the lower end of your esophagus and reduce reflux. The surgeon performs the operation at a hospital. You receive general anesthesia and can leave the hospital in 1 to 3 days. Most people return to their usual daily activities in 2 to 3 weeks.

Endoscopic techniques, such as endoscopic sewing and radiofrequency, help control GERD in a small number of people. Endoscopic sewing uses small stitches to tighten your sphincter muscle. Radiofrequency creates heat lesions, or sores, that help tighten your sphincter muscle. A surgeon performs both operations using an endoscope at a hospital or an outpatient center, and you receive general anesthesia.

The results for endoscopic techniques may not be as good as those for fundoplication. Doctors don't use endoscopic techniques often.

2. 337 Great Tips For Acid Reflux and Heartburn Relief

Is acid reflux a huge obstacle in your life? Would you like to put it to rest? Do you want to learn how to deal with the symptoms? Continue reading to find out some great advice about the topic at hand.

1. If you notice that spicy foods cause you problems, do not eat anything with peppers or chilies in them. This will help to prevent heartburn. At the very least, reduce the frequency with which you eat these items. You should notice an immediate difference in the way that you feel.

2. Never, ever, EVER lie down after you eat! Even if you have only had a few bites, you may find that food comes back to haunt you in short order if you lie down. Eat all meals at least two hours before lying down for a nap or overnight to ensure that acid doesn't sneak back up your esophagus.

3. Many pregnant women suffer from acid reflux. The space taken up by the baby pushes the

stomach and acid upward. You can avoid acid reflux by eating foods low in fat and acid. If this fails, certain types of tea can help buffer stomach acid without causing harm to your baby.

4. Keep chewing gum handy. When you chew gum, it not only freshens your breath, but it causes you to salivate. This helps wash acid down your esophagus and back into your stomach, where it belongs. When choosing a flavor, avoid citrus and mint. Mint can cause your esophageal sphincter to relax, and citrus is high in acid.

5. Stop smoking if you are trying to rid yourself of issues with acid reflux. Many people do not know this, but smoking causes the muscles in the esophagus to relax. This can create some of the symptoms associated with acid reflux, so quit if you are trying to make things better.

6. When your symptoms are at their worst, mix 1 teaspoon of regular baking soda with eight ounces of water. Drink this slowly, one sip at a time, until your symptoms subside. Do NOT do this every day as baking soda contains a great deal of sodium which can lead to a myriad of other health problems.

7. When you want to reach for a natural treatment for heartburn, consider licorice. You need to choose DGL licorice which doesn't contain glycyrrhizic acid and therefore will not cause hypertension. Chewable tablets are your best bet before meals, and they can be found affordably at natural food retailers and health supplement shops.

8. Keep a food journal if you suffer from acid reflux. Anyone who deals with acid reflux has certain foods that causes the onset of this problem. After figuring out your triggers, you can avoid these foods.

9. If you have acid reflux symptoms during the day and at night, gum might solve the problem. Chewing gum helps you produce more saliva. Saliva is a natural neutralizer of stomach acid. If you can, try chewing gum even through the night to try to decrease your level of discomfort through the night and into the morning.

10. Avoid alcohol if you suffer from acid reflux. Alcohol causes overproduction of stomach acid, which leads to the deterioration of your stomach lining as well as acid reflux. Keep your alcohol intake to a minimum, or none at all, to avoid the symptoms of acid reflux.

11. It is known that smoking is bad for your health, but did you also know that smoking can have an affect on acid reflux? When you smoke, more stomach acid is produced, digestion is slowed down, and less saliva is produced. Smoking also causes the sphincter of the esophagus to weaken, making acid reflux occur.

12. Learn stress coping techniques. Being stressed out can cause you to tense up your body and this causes you to contract some, or all, of your stomach muscles, causing acid reflux symptoms. Learn how to better handle stressful situations and you'll find out you may have much less stomach troubles.

13. If your acid reflux is severe, then the importance of not lying flat on your back cannot be stressed enough. Therefore, whenever you sleep, you need to keep your entire upper body slightly elevated. You cannot just add more pillows to lay your head on because this just elevates your head, which is not enough. Place wooden blocks or bricks underneath your mattress can significantly help in relieving your acid reflux symptoms.

14. Do not eat large meals right before you go to bed at night. Avoid eating three hours before bedtime. Laying down with food in your stomach will cause the acid to burn your esophagus.

15. See a physician right away if you have bloody stools or are vomiting. You may have a very serious problem that needs to be addressed. Sometimes, acid reflux may stem from a problem that is already there.

16. Are you suffering with the painful heartburn associated with acid reflux? A natural solution to alleviate this pain can be found in your kitchen. Juicing can help give you relief. Cabbage juice, carrot juice and aloe vera juice are nutrient sources that provide relief. Since these juices sooth the esophagus, they can bring you safe relief.

17. Acid reflux prevention can be done through eating smaller meals and eating more frequently. Meals with larger portions cause unnecessary pressure to be created on the LES or lower esophageal sphincter, which causes the reflux. Try to limit your portion sizes, eating around 5 small meals and properly chewing your food.

18. Exercising your abdominal muscles could cause acid reflux. You should get some exercise after eating to make digestion easier, but going for a walk is enough. Avoid lifting things or putting any kind of pressure on your abs. If your job requires you to be active immediately after your lunch break, choose your foods carefully.

19. Try to avoid drinking anything while you eat. When you drink, your stomach fills up and expands, which can cause distension. This puts pressure on the sphincter at the bottom of the esophagus, sometimes causing food to pass back up through it. When this happens, acid reflux has begun, as will your suffering.

20. Acid reflux can be a normal reaction of eating too much or too quickly! If you've been experiencing the effects of acid reflux lately, change your eating habits. Improve the content of your meals by adding healthier choices and take the time to chew your food well. Your digestive track will appreciate it and you should not suffer with acid reflux so much

21. To help avoid acid reflux, take your time and chew your food slowly. This technique helps you to avoid overeating. When you overeat, food is pressed in the top of your stomach; thus, it

allows stomach acids to build up in you esophagus. For best results, eat small meals often.

22. Eating large portions is a huge cause of acid reflux in a lot of people. When the stomach is too full, it puts too much pressure on the muscles in your stomach. It is better to eat five smaller meals instead of three larger ones. You will eat the same amount, but you will reduce the amount of acid your body produces.

23. Contracting the abdominal muscles can make food that is in your stomach to make its way back into the esophagus. This is why you need to wait until at least one hour after eating before you attempt to do any physical exercise. You should also avoid any other types of physical exertion directly after meals.

24. Wait to exercise after you eat. If you put off your exercise by at least an hour, the food will have a better chance to digest. Physical exertion right after you eat could cause the food to move back up toward the esophagus. This could be very uncomfortable and hard to fight.

25. Try to avoid eating chocolate if you have issues with acid reflux. The caffeine and alkaloids that

are contained in chocolate tend to disagree with people that have this problem. If you must have chocolate, each it in small quantities and opt for a darker chocolate since it has antioxidants.

26. Drinking a large amount of liquid while eating can lead to acid reflux. You may not think about it, but liquids also add to the volume of food in your stomach. When the volume of food is too great, it overpowers your body's resources to keep food in your stomach. Limit the amount of liquid you drink while eating, or only drink between meals.

27. Everyone has a few foods that cause them to experience acid reflux. Limit your consumption of trigger foods to help prevent acid reflux. A few foods that frequently cause problems are tomatoes, milk, alcohol, acidic juices, coffee or spicy foods.

28. Exercise often if you want to improve your condition. The key to this is moderate. Extreme exercise can actually interfere with digestion, worsening acid reflux symptoms. However, moderate exercise reduces reflux. Such exercises work to keep you in an upright position, allowing gravity to aid digestion. You will also lose weight by exercising, therefore reducing heartburn.

29. If you are overweight or obese and you have acid reflux disease, you should do your best to lose weight. When you are overweight, organs surrounding the stomach could actually push into the stomach, causing too much acid to form. It could even weaken your esophagus, making it more likely for acid to come up.

30. Try to eat slowly. Eating too fast will cause acid reflux to strike. If you find that you have trouble with this, make an effort to take a bite and then put your utensil down. This will ensure that you don't put too much food in your mouth at any given time.

31. Tell your doctor about all of the medications that you are taking at the moment, as there can be a relation between them and your acid reflux. Medications can worsen your symptoms and reduce the effectiveness of your stomach and esophageal function. A drug-free lifestyle may be the answer to your acid reflux.

32. Gluten is a frequent cause of acid reflux. Foods with gluten, such as oats, barely or wheat, need to be avoided by people who have acid reflux. You may find a small amount of grains helpful.

33. Stick to raw foods instead of processed foods if you want to help speed up your digestive functionality and reduce acid reflux symptoms. Raw foods are healthier and are easier for your stomach to process effectively. This can help you live a healthier lifestyle that is filled with the nutrients that you require.

34. Do not lie down less than two hours after every meal in order to avoid acid reflux. This is because gravity is a simple method of limiting acid reflux. Listen to your body. The period of time you must remain upright is an individual matter. It also depends on what you have eaten.

35. Although not always the case, tight clothing can sometimes cause acid reflux. If a belt or waistband seems tight, try loosening your clothing to relieve the discomfort. When too much pressure is put on your midsection, gastric acid can be forced from the stomach and upward into your esophagus, creating the burning sensation.

36. Dealing with acid reflux is no laughing matter. The suffering those who have this condition deal with daily can be debilitating. Thankfully, there are some options out there which will help you tame your acid reflux once and for all. Keep

reading for some simple tips which will help to change your life forever.

37. You may need to change your diet if you suffer from acid reflux disease. Sugary and processed foods increase the amount of acid that is produced in your stomach, the cause of acid reflux disease. Fruits and vegetables are great foods to eat that do not cause or worsen acid reflux.

38. Pregnant women often start developing acid reflux. The baby can puts pressure on the stomach and the acid will spread to the esophagus. When pregnant it is a good idea to avoid trouble foods, and eat low fat foods to prevent problems. If this isn't helping, you can drink some teas that are safe for the baby and that can neutralize stomach acid.

39. Keep chewing gum handy. When you chew gum, it not only freshens your breath, but it causes you to salivate. This helps wash acid down your esophagus and back into your stomach, where it belongs. When choosing a flavor, avoid citrus and mint. Mint can cause your esophageal sphincter to relax, and citrus is high in acid.

40. Sometimes, there is nothing that can be done to prevent acid reflux disease. This is why you need to learn of what you can do when an attack occurs. Try drinking cold milk or eating some cracker or bread. These remedies help by reducing the amount of acid that comes up through the esophagus.

41. Chew cinnamon gum after meals. The chewing causes more saliva to be generated in the mouth and throat. Saliva is formulated to help balance the mix of acid in your stomach. Chewing gum also causes a person to swallow more often, which cleans the throat of acids that come up from the stomach. If not cinnamon gum, fruit flavors work as well. Mint relaxes your esophageal sphincter, so avoid it in gum.

42. You should always take your time to eat slowly. Enjoy your food and find a peaceful and quiet environment where you can eat. If you feel stressed, take a few minutes to relax before beginning to eat your food. Digestion will be much easier if you are relaxed and take your time.

43. Try to drink mostly in between meals if you suffer from acid reflux. When your stomach is full of food an liquid, the lower esophageal sphincter is under constant pressure. This can

cause it to allow the food and acid in your stomach to come back up into your esophagus and destroy the lining within.

44. Beans are a food that can worsen acid reflux disease. Stomach acids form due to foods that are rough on the stomach and beans fall into this category. This tends to go for all kinds of beans, so as healthy as they may be, you may need to totally cut them out of your diet.

45. Stop smoking to help with your reflux symptoms. Smoking can increase your chances of developing GERD too. It slows down digestion, boots stomach acid, and reduces the production of saliva. Without a higher production of saliva, you don't have a great defense against the stomach acid. It also harms the esophagus, weakens your LES muscle and weakens your whole digestive system, which can contribute to acid reflux.

46. Avoid foods that trigger acid reflux. These include alcohol, caffeinated beverages such as coffee, tea and soda, fatty foods, spicy foods and acidic foods such as tomatoes. When you are suffering from acid reflux, eat a variety of fruits and vegetables, lean proteins such as broiled fish and chicken and enriched grains.

47. If acid reflux is a serious problem for you, examine your typical posture. Although sitting up

straight will not cure your symptoms, it will improve them. When you are hunched over, you contort inner organs and muscles in unnatural positions and that can worsen your acid reflux problem. Sit completely upright and relax, for ease of symptoms and less back pain too.

48. Avoid lying down after you eat for at least two hours. Instead, get up and walk around to help your digestive tract work properly. The first two hours after eating is the perfect time to do the dishes, clean the house and go for a walk. Additionally, if your acid reflux flares up while you sleep, use risers to slightly elevate the head of your bed to help avoid stomach acids from going into your esophagus.

49. Coffee and tea can trigger acid reflux, so try to avoid them. Both of these beverages are typically high in caffeine, and this is often even true if you choose decaffeinated varieties. Try to limit your consumption of both beverages whenever possible, and instead, make a healthy choice, like drinking water.

50. If you are not too keen on the idea of taking medication to control your acid reflux, there is still something you can do to. Many foods can naturally help you combat your acid reflux.

Herbal licorice has the ability to naturally coat your stomach with a protective gel when it is taken in tincture or tea form.

51. Stay away from extremely greasy food in order to combat the onset of an acid reflux attack. Many fast food products such as crispy chicken sandwiches, french fries, or hamburgers can cause this. It is best to stick with meat that has less fat and has been prepared in a healthier way such as turkey and grilled chicken.

52. Are you suffering from acid reflux due to being pregnant? If so, then you need to determine the cause as soon as possible. Something as silly or simple as drinking water after 7 in the evening could be the trigger. By learning what is causing your acid reflux, you can stop it in its tracks.

53. Slow down! When you eat more slowly, your body is able to keep up with what is being deposited in your stomach. This means that it will know that it is full when it truly is full, and you will eat less. If you overeat, you'll find your acid reflux goes crazy.

54. When your symptoms are at their worst, mix 1 teaspoon of regular baking soda with eight ounces of water. Drink this slowly, one sip at a

time, until your symptoms subside. Do NOT do
this every day as baking soda contains a great
deal of sodium which can lead to a myriad of
other health problems.

55. Loosen up if you've been dealing with too much
acid reflux. Your clothing, that is. Tight pants,
close-fitting shirts or pantyhose can make
symptoms of acid reflux much worse. If you can,
put a robe on or other over-sized and very comfy
clothes and take it easy. Your symptoms should
at least be somewhat alleviated.

56. Limit the amount of liquid you consume with all
your meals. Too much liquid can cause the
stomach to become much too full, which
increases your chances of suffering from acid
reflux symptoms. You should only allow yourself
to have small sips of water in between your bites
of food.

57. Chew a stick of gum if you feel like your acid
reflux issue is not under control at night. A stick
of gum can increase the amount of saliva that
you have in your mouth, which can help push
down the acid that is getting into your esophagus
from your stomach.

58. A lozenge containing slippery elm may give you some relief. This lozenge can provide a shield and extra liner to your digestive tract. This lozenge also works to prevent the cough that acid reflux can cause. You can find them at any health food stores and natural food stores near you.

59. Include plenty of high fiber foods into your diet. High fiber foods absorb the fats which will limit the effects of acid reflux. Good choices of high fiber foods should include natural grains such as wheat bread, brown rice and starchy vegetables like potatoes and beans. Incorporate some high fiber choices into each meal for best results.

60. One of the best things you can do if you suffer from acid reflux is to lose a few pounds. Obesity is a huge contributor to acid reflux and heartburn. If you are at a healthy weight, statistics show that you are less than half as likely to suffer from acid reflux as people who are overweight. This is a great reason to shed some pounds.

61. Learn to manage the stress in your life if you've been experiencing frequent symptoms of acid reflux. A nervous stomach will certainly exacerbate your problem and make diagnosing

the real causes difficult. Eat in a calm environment and savor each bite. Forget about the stress in your life at least during the meal; it's better for your mind and body.

62. One of the worst things you can do if you suffer from acid reflux is to lie down after a meal. It is very important that for at least two hours after you eat, you do not lie flat on your back or stomach. It is best if you stand up and walk a little bit. This will help get your stomach juices flowing in the right direction.

63. Did you know that acid reflux, when untreated, can lead to ulcers? You can have perforations of both the stomach and esophageal lining, leading to intense pain. When your heartburn seems to have kicked up a notch, talk to your doctor to get the right tests done to rule out this complication.

64. Stay away from fast food if you want to prevent acid reflux from happening during the day. Fast food contains a lot of fat, which can build up in your stomach and cause acid to build up. Eat healthy meals if you want to feel fresh, energized and free of pain.

65. Are you overweight? Being too heavy could cause your stomach acid to go back up into your esophagus. Therefore, making an effort to eat right and exercise daily will help you with your symptoms. If necessary, speak with your doctor to see if they have any advice or suggestions for you.

66. Avoid eating spicy foods in the evening if you suffer from acid reflux. Spicy foods includes jalepenos, peppers and Mexican foods. Spicy foods also can cause indigestion and dry skin on top of your acid reflux, so this makes things worse.

67. Cut down on the amount of coffee that you consume if you want to eliminate GERD symptoms. There is nothing wrong with having a small cup of coffee in the morning, but if you are consuming three to four large lattes every day, that is asking for acid reflux issues.

68. If you are big into exercising, be moderate about your high-impact exercises. Major exertion in these hardcore fitness regimens can actually make your acid reflux worse. Instead, mix it up and get some time with more moderate fitness routines. A great choice is a long walk at a medium speed.

69. Knowing your triggers is truly the only way to totally conquer your acid reflux. If you eat tomatoes and experience discomfort, stop eating tomatoes. Keep a meal diary tracking everything you eat and drink and a mood diary which logs how you feel, then compare them to see what your problem areas are.

70. Acid reflux can be a normal reaction of eating too much or too quickly! If you've been experiencing the effects of acid reflux lately, change your eating habits. Improve the content of your meals by adding healthier choices and take the time to chew your food well. Your digestive track will appreciate it and you should not suffer with acid reflux so much

71. Exercise is a good way to stop acid reflux. Through exercise, you can lose weight, which will put less pressure on the stomach and reduce the severity and occurrence of heartburn and acid reflux. The key is to use moderate, low impact exercises. Intense exercises can cause reflux through excessive agitation. Try to avoid drinking sports drinks and eating food before exercising, as these can cause reflux as well.

72. Our acid reflux can be triggered by specific foods. Common trigger foods include fried

foods, caffeinated beverages, alcohol, and chocolate. Citrus fruits and acidic vegetables like tomatoes are also well known culprits. Different people have different triggers, and it will take time to learn which ones affect you. If you want to be completely safe, just avoid these things.

73. Stay upright after eating. It can be quite helpful if you stay sitting or standing for at least two to three hours after you eat a meal. This will give your food time to digest and help keep your acid reflux symptoms down to a minimum. If you must lie down, do your best to elevate your body above your waist.

74. Acid reflux symptoms can be aggravated by vigorous exercise after meals. Contractions of the lower stomach during exercise can cause undigested food to be forced upwards in the esophagus. Wait for a couple of hours before you work out.

75. There are many over-the-counter medications you can take for acid reflux. They are called antacids and they work by stopping excess acid production. Just be aware that no one medication works for everyone. If you try one and it is not effective for you, keep trying others until you find the right one for you.

76. The food you consume each day will make a difference in your reflux. Avoiding acidic foods, peppers, greasy foods and alcoholic beverages could help. These foods and drinks could be causing the problem. Also, avoid eating less than three hours before you bed time. Going to bed with a full stomach could make for a rough night and morning.

77. Shed excess pounds to decrease the impact of acid reflux. Obesity can put excess pressure on your stomach. Even if you lose 10 percent of the current weight, you can reduce your symptoms. If you are trying to lose weight, make sure you use a sensible eating plan.

78. Limit the amount of drinks you have when you eat. Beverages can add volume to the food that you digest and increase how distended your stomach is. Having a full stomach puts some pressure on your LES or lower esophageal sphincter, which is responsible for keeping food from getting back into the esophagus. This increases your chances for having reflux. To lower chances, take small sips when eating and try drinking your beverages between meals instead of during meals.

79. Changing the time you exercise can help decrease the amount of acid reflux symptoms you get. Contracting your abdominal muscles can force any food in your stomach to go back into your esophagus. It is best to wait about an hour after you exercise to take part in any sort of exercise.

80. Learn to manage the stress in your life if you've been experiencing frequent symptoms of acid reflux. A nervous stomach will certainly exacerbate your problem and make diagnosing the real causes difficult. Eat in a calm environment and savor each bite. Forget about the stress in your life at least during the meal; it's better for your mind and body.

81. One of the worst things you can do if you suffer from acid reflux is to lie down after a meal. It is very important that for at least two hours after you eat, you do not lie flat on your back or stomach. It is best if you stand up and walk a little bit. This will help get your stomach juices flowing in the right direction.

82. If you smoke, you need to quit. Obviously, there are many reasons why you should quit, but if you suffer from acid reflux, this is yet another reason. Smoking slows down your digestion and reduces

your saliva production, which worsens acid reflux symptoms. In addition, smoking harms your LES muscle, further worsening your acid reflux. Quitting this terrible habit can significantly improve your acid reflux, not to mention all the other benefits.

83. Your body weight can play a major role in your stomach issues. Having extra fat in your mid-section puts extra added pressure on your stomach and increases acid reflux symptoms. If you have some weight to lose, losing it can help you cut down on acid reflux incidences. Living a healthier lifestyle can help you feel better in more ways than one.

84. If acid reflux is a serious problem for you, examine your typical posture. Although sitting up straight will not cure your symptoms, it will improve them. When you are hunched over, you contort inner organs and muscles in unnatural positions and that can worsen your acid reflux problem. Sit completely upright and relax, for ease of symptoms and less back pain too.

85. Slow down! When you eat more slowly, your body is able to keep up with what is being deposited in your stomach. This means that it will know that it is full when it truly is full, and

you will eat less. If you overeat, you'll find your acid reflux goes crazy.

86. Turn to aloe vera juice for a soothing way to heal the damage acid reflux can cause. It reduces inflammation in the esophagus and the lining of the stomach itself. All you need is a half a cup before a meal to aid in your digestive regeneration, but remember that it is also a laxative!

87. When you complete your meal, do not lie down on your back or stomach. This position uses gravity to build up acid in your stomach, which is one of the main reasons why you get acid reflux and heartburn. Walk around your home or do the dishes after you eat to prevent this from happening.

88. Medications that are available over the counter at a drugstore or pharmacy will only temporarily mask acid reflux disease symptoms with not much effectiveness. If you find yourself using these products with increasing regularity, you should consult a doctor. They can prescribe stronger prescription medications that prevent acid reflux from occurring.

89. Don't lie down after eating. When you recline, your digestion slows down. Remaining in a seated position allows you to bypass the unpleasant effects of acid reflux.

90. When working out to help your acid reflux, be cautious of what and when you consume food and beverages. Eating too soon or eating and drinking the wrong things can negate the positive effects of exercise for your reflux. You should wait at least two hours after a workout to eat. Don't drink sports drinks since their acidity can trigger your reflux.

91. Skip the antacid. An antacid is fine if you only suffer from acid reflux occasionally, however more frequent sufferers should look for better treatment options. An antacid is only a temporary fix, working to mask the pain. It does nothing to treat the underlying cause of the problem. Using antacids too frequently can even cause your stomach to start producing more acid in response.

92. Try drinking less during a meal to help with your acid reflux. Liquids can cause food to expand in your body, and they increase the volume of foods inside of your body. Instead, consider eating your meals first, and then enjoy your

beverage about fifteen minutes after your meal is through.

93. Have an early dinner. Eating too close to bedtime is a prime cause of acid reflux. If your stomach is still digesting your dinner when you retire, the combination of increased stomach activity and a horizontal position is a recipe for disaster. Try to eat dinner a minimum of three hours before bed.

94. Sleep at least 8 hours at night to help prevent acid reflux in your life. A good amount of rest during the night can help your body to recuperate from the day and get back to 100%. This will aid in reducing the acid in your body, which is a catalyst for acid reflux.

95. Stop smoking to help with your reflux symptoms. Smoking can increase your chances of developing GERD too. It slows down digestion, boots stomach acid, and reduces the production of saliva. Without a higher production of saliva, you don't have a great defense against the stomach acid. It also harms the esophagus, weakens your LES muscle and weakens your whole digestive system, which can contribute to acid reflux.

96. When you experience acid reflux, you should try taking some ginger. You could eat it or put it in your tea or certain foods if you would like. For ages, ginger has been used as an anti-inflammatory and has also been down to reduce gastrointestinal conditions, acid reflux disease includes.

97. An excellent method of reducing your acid reflux symptoms is consuming your meals as slowly as possible. After you have taken a few bites of food, put down your fork or spoon and rest so that your stomach can properly digest. Allow yourself to actually enjoy what you are eating! Don't eat too much during a single meal and stop eating when you're full instead of stuffed.

98. If you have acid reflux, there are some natural solutions that will help reduce some of your heartburn. If you begin using calcium supplements, you can start alleviating heartburn. The reason why calcium can reduce, or even prevent, heartburn is because it strengthens the lower esophageal sphincter (LES). Since calcium isn't an anti-acid, it won't provide fast relief. However, over time, it will provide long-term relief.

99. Chewing gum can help with the symptoms of acid reflux. Gum helps produce saliva in the mouth and throat, which helps clean the esophagus. This keeps the acid from building up and causing uncomfortable symptoms. Chew sugar-free gums like Trident or Dentine to prevent tooth decay or any other dental issues.

100.   You might suffer from occasional acid reflux and need some relief, but not necessarily from a daily medication. There are many great antacids available over the counter that work quickly for the occasional acid reflux. These medications can be taken before a particular meal, or even after once the acid reflux has already started.

101.   Watch your intake of food right before it is time for bed. Eating within two hours of the time you will be laying down for the evening can lead to acid build up in your digestive system and cause reflux problems. Instead, limit your after dinner snacks as much as possible.

102.   When you are done eating a meal, prevent acid reflux by chewing on some gum. More saliva is produced when you chew some gum. The more saliva that is produced during digestion, the less acid is produced, in turn, preventing acid reflux from occurring. Ideally, you should chew on sugar-free gum.

103. It is a good idea to raise the head of your bed if you have been experiencing acid reflux issues frequently. When you are lying flat, it gives the stomach contents an easier way of refluxing. You should raise the mattress about 6-8 inches in order to get the best results.

104. In order to ameliorate the pain and discomfort of acid reflux, consider breaking your daily food intake into five or so smaller meals instead of three main ones. This helps prevent you from overloading your digestive system at any one time, making acids work more effectively in smaller amounts. You will soon start to notice a real change in your symptoms for the better.

105. Treat your acid reflux symptoms by hydrating yourself. Increase your intake of water. Of course, water hydrates you as you work out. Additionally, it helps you digest your food. Water can dilute the acid present in your stomach and make acid reflux less painful.

106. Try popping a few pieces of chewing gum into your mouth every time you are feeling the symptoms of acid reflux. This will cause the body to produce a much larger amount of saliva

than it does on a regular basis, and this will help neutralize the acid inside of the stomach.

107.   There is a drug called phenylalanine and it is found inside of most over-the-counter antacids. If you have acid reflux and you also have mental retardation and/or seizures, you should not take them. This is because the phenylalanine will make you more prone to having seizures. Talk to your doctor about other options.

108.   If you are overweight, your recurring acid reflux problem could be caused by your extra pounds. Focus on losing some weight in your midsection to reduce the pressure on your stomach and make digestion easier. You can easily get in shape by doing some abs and adopting a healthier diet.

109.   Try to drink mostly in between meals if you suffer from acid reflux. When your stomach is full of food an liquid, the lower esophageal sphincter is under constant pressure. This can cause it to allow the food and acid in your stomach to come back up into your esophagus and destroy the lining within.

110.   Speak to a doctor if you feel like your acid reflux is not improving from the antacids that

you are taking on a daily basis. Sometimes, you may need a serious form of medication that you doctor can prescribe, which can improve your symptoms. A professional's diagnosis may be the solution to your acid reflux issues.

111.   Were you aware that the acid in food really does not affect the pH balance of the food? Some seemingly acidic foods (e.g. lemons) may be quite alkaline when digested. The pH levels in foods can be quite confusing. However, if you have acid reflux, you need to educate yourself on food pH.

112.   Avoid lying down after you've eaten. If you are prone to acid reflux, avoid laying flat for at least two hours after a snack or meal. Standing or walking can actually help your gastric juices start flowing properly. When you do go to sleep, try keeping the upper portion of your body elevated using a foam wedge or some books under the mattress or propping up your legs with blocks or books.

113.   Try relaxing. If you eat when stressed, it can lead to acid reflux. Truly relaxing after a meal using deep breathing exercises or meditation can help cut down on acid reflux. Never lie down; stay up!

114.   There are lots of potential trigger foods that can cause you heartburn and acid reflux. Try to avoid these foods. The usual suspects are fatty fried foods, caffeinated drinks, chocolate, alcohol, citrus juices and fruits, spicy foods, tomatoes and beverages with lots of carbonation. If you just avoid these foods, you will eliminate many symptoms.

115.   If you smoke, you need to quit. Obviously, there are many reasons why you should quit, but if you suffer from acid reflux, this is yet another reason. Smoking slows down your digestion and reduces your saliva production, which worsens acid reflux symptoms. In addition, smoking harms your LES muscle, further worsening your acid reflux. Quitting this terrible habit can significantly improve your acid reflux, not to mention all the other benefits.

116.   When people have acid reflux, chewing cinnamon gum can offer them some relief. Chewing causes saliva to be produced, neutralizing acid. You will also swallow more saliva and keep the acid down. This increased swallowing carries the acid back to the stomach and keeps it from causing heartburn.

117.   Get medium-level exercise into your daily routine. Exercises such as walking for two miles can really help your digestion. As an added benefit, it can also help you lose weight which can again help your acid reflux issues. It's a win on both ways! Steer clear of high-level exercise though, as it can actually cause your acid reflux to spike.

118.   To reduce the risk of acid reflux, try not to drink beverages with your meal. Drinking will add volume to the food in your stomach. This causes more pressure on the esophageal sphincter, which in turn causes acid reflux. You should drink between two meals instead of during your meals.

119.   Stay away from acidic foods. They can both cause and exacerbate acid reflux. While this is by no means a comprehensive list, try to avoid oranges, tomatoes, grapefruit and vinegar. If you can't cut them out of your diet completely, at least try to avoid eating them in the evenings, so acid reflux doesn't strike when it is time for bed.

120.   It is important that you don't eat too quickly if you suffer from acid reflux. The slower you eat, the better! Not only will it allow you to begin to break down the food in your stomach, it will ensure that you feel full when you really are full,

something that doesn't happen if you eat too quickly.

121.   Keep a diet diary. Everyone is different, and which foods will trigger your acid reflux may not be the same as mine. Write down how you feel before, during and after each meal, and include a list of what you eat and drink all day. After a month, you should have a clearer picture of which foods cause you the most grief.

122.   Try eating your meals slower. Due to the extremely fast-paced world we live in, we tend to always be in a hurry. This carries over to our eating, causing us to eat way too fast. This increases the odds that we will overeat, which can cause acid reflux. Instead, take your time while eating. Thoroughly chew your food, and put down your fork after every few bites. Stop eating once you feel comfortable, not stuffed.

123.   Contracting the abdominal muscles can make food that is in your stomach to make its way back into the esophagus. This is why you need to wait until at least one hour after eating before you attempt to do any physical exercise. You should also avoid any other types of physical exertion directly after meals.

124.   If you drop excess pounds, you may find relief from reflux. Obesity is one of the leading causes. Just losing a small amount of weight can help. Don't crash diet to lose weight, instead start eating less and exercising more.

125.   There is a drug called phenylalanine and it is found inside of most over-the-counter antacids. If you have acid reflux and you also have mental retardation and/or seizures, you should not take them. This is because the phenylalanine will make you more prone to having seizures. Talk to your doctor about other options.

126.   Drinking a large amount of liquid while eating can lead to acid reflux. You may not think about it, but liquids also add to the volume of food in your stomach. When the volume of food is too great, it overpowers your body's resources to keep food in your stomach. Limit the amount of liquid you drink while eating, or only drink between meals.

127.   Try moderate exercise that keeps you upright, such as walking. Exercise like this can help lessen the acid reflux effects, for a variety of reasons. First, keeping upright aids in proper digestion. It also contributes to weight loss, which helps to prevent reflux. Exercising is

important, but working out too intensely could make your acid reflux worse, for instance, if you contract your abdominal muscles after a meal.

128.   Lose weight by going to the gym and performing cardiovascular exercises if you want to limit your acid reflux symptoms. If you are overweight, you will have a better chance of acid reflux building in your stomach and causing heartburn. Exercising can help with your heartburn and improve your health at the same time.

129.   If you are overweight, your recurring acid reflux problem could be caused by your extra pounds. Focus on losing some weight in your midsection to reduce the pressure on your stomach and make digestion easier. You can easily get in shape by doing some abs and adopting a healthier diet.

130.   Losing some weight can help with your acid reflux. Being overweight can contribute to heartburn. The extra pounds can cause excess pressure on the stomach making the LES or lower esophageal sphincter relax causing backflow. Extra body fat can also release some chemicals that interfere with normal digestion.

Losing a few pounds can relieve many of these symptoms and keep heartburn to a minimum.

131.   Slippery elm lozenge are a good natural remedy to try. These are derived from the bark of the slippery elm tree. They are natural and work to provide a soothing coating for your throat and internal organs. They also help to calm coughing and soothe irritation. Health food stores are the most likely place to find slippery elm lozenges.

132.   Don't rush your eating. When you eat to fast, you can trigger acid reflux. Instead really take time to enjoy your meal as much as you can. Put your fork down every so often and let your body digest throughout the sitting. Don't eat to being overly full. You'll be much less likely to have issues.

133.   Quit smoking immediately to prevent acid reflux from occurring. Smoking cigarettes can increase the nicotine content that enters your body, which can damage your esophagus. A damaged esophagus can lead to more acid buildup in your body and trigger acid reflux episodes. Also, smoking will help you to live a healthier lifestyle and reduce esophageal cancer.

134.   For those who suffer from acid reflux, chewing cinnamon gum right after eating can help. Chewing stimulates salivation which helps with digestion by neutralizing stomach acids. Chewing gum makes you swallow more, too. This pushes stomach acid down into the stomach, instead of allowing it to come up into your esophagus.

135.   Stay away from acidic foods. They can both cause and exacerbate acid reflux. While this is by no means a comprehensive list, try to avoid oranges, tomatoes, grapefruit and vinegar. If you can't cut them out of your diet completely, at least try to avoid eating them in the evenings, so acid reflux doesn't strike when it is time for bed.

136.   The fattier a food is, the worse the acid reflux becomes. Foods high in fat relax the esophageal sphincter so much that it allows acid to come up. Fatty foods cause weight gain, which also adds to acid reflux problems. Learn to make good nutritional choices.

137.   Limit your liquid intake with meals if you're prone to acid reflux. Even healthy beverages like water can fill up your stomach fast, creating conditions that are conducive to acid reflux. Sip your beverage conservatively and never gulp it

down. Wait a half an hour after a big meal to enjoy quenching your thirst.

138.   For quick relief, pick up cinnamon flavored gum. When you chew gum, your salivary glands pick up the pace which can help neutralize stomach acid. On top of that, you'll swallow more and help clear the acid out of your esophagus. Lastly, choosing non-mint and non-citrus flavors ensures you don't trigger your acid reflux.

139.   If you suffer with acid reflux, understand how gravity can work in your favor. Sitting upright will help keep food and fluids down after meals, so keep yourself straight. Avoid lying down or even slightly reclining in your favorite chair as this will exacerbate reflux symptoms quickly. Try going for a short and healthy walk instead!

140.   Do you suffer from respiratory problems? Do you have a chronic couch or wheeze often? If so, it could be an acid reflux problem. Heartburn could cause these symptoms. Your doctor might suggest a pH test. This procedure is done on an outpatient basis over the course of 24 hours and can determine if reflux is a problem.

141.   If you are active and experiencing acid reflux, you may just need to make one simple change. Enjoy a tall glass of water. Your body will be more hydrated. Water also facilitates digestion. You decrease and dilute your stomach acid by increasing your water intake.

142.   The food you consume each day will make a difference in your reflux. Avoiding acidic foods, peppers, greasy foods and alcoholic beverages could help. These foods and drinks could be causing the problem. Also, avoid eating less than three hours before you bed time. Going to bed with a full stomach could make for a rough night and morning.

143.   While eating your meals, limit your beverage consumption. Although this may sound silly, drinking lots of beverages during your meals can actually cause acid reflux. This is because liquids increase the volume of food in your stomach. When your stomach is full, the lower esophageal sphincter has more pressure placed upon it. This muscle prevents food from coming up through your esophagus, which prevents acid reflux. You need to protect your lower esophageal sphincter as much as possible.

144.   If you suffer with acid reflux, don't lay down after eating. When you lie down, your body will not digest the food you've just eaten correctly. By staying upright, you can avoid acid from going into your esophagus.

145.   Try to eliminate stress caused by work, school or relationship issues. Stress produces stomach acid, which in turn can cause inflammation and heartburn pain. Identify the cause of your stress and get it under control ASAP.

146.   For children who have acid reflux disease, the only thing that may work for them is time. When a person is younger, their digestive systems have not yet matured. This makes it easier for acid to produce, thus, increase acid reflux symptoms. Once they get older, the problem should go away.

147.   Smaller portion sizes will help you control your acid reflux. If you eat a little less at each meal, you shouldn't have as much trouble with heartburn. You could also try eating five or six small meals, instead of three large meals each day if you want to make a difference.

148. Changing the time you exercise can help decrease the amount of acid reflux symptoms you get. Contracting your abdominal muscles can force any food in your stomach to go back into your esophagus. It is best to wait about an hour after you exercise to take part in any sort of exercise.

149. Tomatoes may be a tasty and healthy food, but it is not good for those who have acid reflux disease. The amount of acid found in tomatoes is astonishing. If you have acid reflux disease, you should avoid tomatoes and any products that contain them if you want to reduce symptoms.

150. Stay away from extremely greasy food in order to combat the onset of an acid reflux attack. Many fast food products such as crispy chicken sandwiches, french fries, or hamburgers can cause this. It is best to stick with meat that has less fat and has been prepared in a healthier way such as turkey and grilled chicken.

151. Avoid eating spicy foods in the evening if you suffer from acid reflux. Mexican food and hot peppers are perfect examples. Eating spicy foods can trigger reflux and cause indigestion to make your stomach feel even worse.

152.   You need to exercise if you have GERD, but don't overdo it. Losing weight is a huge factor in controlling acid reflux, so go out for a run, play some soccer or go for a swim. That said, don't push your body too hard or you may find your GERD becomes active.

153.   Skinny jeans are the enemy of the acid reflux sufferer! Wearing tight clothes can block up your digestive system, causing you a great deal of pain when acid begins to back up. Go for elastic waistbands until you have your acid reflux under control, then you can consider getting back into your tight fitting pants.

154.   When your symptoms are at their worst, mix 1 teaspoon of regular baking soda with eight ounces of water. Drink this slowly, one sip at a time, until your symptoms subside. Do NOT do this every day as baking soda contains a great deal of sodium which can lead to a myriad of other health problems.

155.   If you smoke and have acid reflux, you may wish to quit. Nicotine causes acid reflux to get worse. Still, don't try to stop immediately. This could cause your acid reflux to get worse, as your body will be going through withdrawal. Quit slowly instead.

156.   Learn your trigger foods. When you know what foods or beverages cause you acid reflux, you can avoid them to keep your symptoms to a minimum. Some foods that often cause symptoms are foods that are fried, fatty, spicy and carbonated drinks. These are just some examples and what bothers someone else, might not bother you.

157.   Certain foods cause acid reflex more than other foods. Keeping a diary of your eating habits can help you understand when acid reflux is at its worst. After you've eaten, if you begin to feel acid reflux symptoms, write down what you ate, what the symptoms are, and how they are affecting you.

158.   A great way to minimize your acid reflux at night is to eat your largest meal of the day at lunch. You want as much of your food to be digested prior to lying down for the night. Rearrange your eating habits to include a big lunch and very small dinner.

159.   Reduce the fat in your diet. Excess fat causes your LES muscle to relax, which delays stomach emptying. As a result, acid reflux is more likely to occur. Therefore, if you consume lots of fried

foods, substitute them for leaner, grilled options. This is not only good for your acid reflux, but also for your overall health.

160.   Slippery elm lozenges are optimal to help with your acid reflux. Slippery elm helps coat your digestive tract. This lozenge can quiet a cough and soothe an upset throat. These can be purchased at many drug stores and at most health and natural food stores.

161.   Don't self diagnose! If you believe you may have this condition due to symptoms, such as stomach discomfort and regurgitation, then you should talk to your doctor. You could have an ulcer or heart problem that just mimics acid reflux. Your doctor may run tests to see if it's acid reflux.

162.   If you smoke, you need to quit. Obviously, there are many reasons why you should quit, but if you suffer from acid reflux, this is yet another reason. Smoking slows down your digestion and reduces your saliva production, which worsens acid reflux symptoms. In addition, smoking harms your LES muscle, further worsening your acid reflux. Quitting this terrible habit can significantly improve your acid reflux, not to mention all the other benefits.

163.   If there are not enough reasons to quit smoking, here is one more. Quitting smoking will greatly reduce the likelihood of contracting GERD. The digestion process is slowed down by smoking and it also increases production of stomach acid. Smoking reduces the production of saliva which is the body's defense against stomach acid.

164.   Keep your stress levels down to prevent flaring up your acid reflux. Stress causes tension and can contract some of your stomach muscles leading to reflux. Watch how you react to emotional or stressful situations to avoid making matters worse in your stomach. Also try keeping your temper below the boiling point to avoid major reflux symptoms.

165.   Avoid foods that trigger acid reflux. These include alcohol, caffeinated beverages such as coffee, tea and soda, fatty foods, spicy foods and acidic foods such as tomatoes. When you are suffering from acid reflux, eat a variety of fruits and vegetables, lean proteins such as broiled fish and chicken and enriched grains.

166.   If you enjoy vigorous exercise, try to avoid participating in activities immediately after a

meal. While some exercise is essential to avoid acid reflux problems, vigorous exercise can upset your digestive system and bring about reflux. Try to space your meals and exercise at least forty five minutes apart, or enjoy less intense exercise immediately following a meal.

167.   Pregnancy may cause acid reflux symptoms. More specifically, a link has been detected between pregnancy and chronic acid reflux. This generally stems from the fact that the weight of the baby is crowding the stomach area. Most of time, the acid reflux symptoms are relieved shortly after the baby has been delivered.

168.   If acid reflux is a serious problem for you, examine your typical posture. Although sitting up straight will not cure your symptoms, it will improve them. When you are hunched over, you contort inner organs and muscles in unnatural positions and that can worsen your acid reflux problem. Sit completely upright and relax, for ease of symptoms and less back pain too.

169.   If you notice that spicy foods cause you problems, do not eat anything with peppers or chilies in them. This will help to prevent heartburn. At the very least, reduce the frequency with which you eat these items. You should

notice an immediate difference in the way that you feel.

170.   Avoid eating spicy foods including those with hot peppers in them. These foods can lead to painful acid reflux after eating, so not eating them can easily remedy your discomfort. Instead, focus on spices which don't lead to pain, such as cinnamon or herbs. They taste great and leave you comfortable post-meal.

171.   Believe it or not, your clothing can affect how often you get acid reflux. Clothing that fits too tightly around the midsection will put excess pressure on the stomach, making reflux occur more often and with more pain. Opt for clothing with a loose fit. Only wear pants and belts that are tight enough to stay up without pressing too hard on the midsection.

172.   Avoid eating large quantities of food that contain a lot of acid. This may cause you to experience heartburn and other acid reflux symptoms. These foods include grapefruit, vinegar, lemons and tomatoes. If you are going to eat these foods, make sure that you are very mindful of the portion size.

173.   To help combat acid reflux, use something to raise up your bed at the head portion only. Use anything from books to bricks to increase the incline. The head of the bed should be six inches more elevated than the bottom of the bed. Elevating your chest helps stop the stomach acid rising in your sleep.

174.   Avoid wearing clothing that is restricting around your abdomen. Wear your belts loosely and avoid pantyhose that are tight if at all possible. These articles could push on your stomach. This pressure on the abdomen could easily lead to heartburn. You may have to do some sit-ups each day to avoid buying new pants and skirts that fit properly.

175.   Particular foods can lead to acid reflux. Limit how many of these items you consume. Things to stay away from are carbonated drinks, acidic juices, milk, coffee, spicy foods and fatty foods.

176.   Try some natural ways to reduce the effects of acid reflux in your body. There are lots of medications that you can take to help with your acid reflux, but why take them if you can control it naturally? Try to eat foods that are alkaline. Foods such as milk, bananas, almonds, tofu and avocados are all alkaline foods.

177.   Try drinking less during a meal to help with your acid reflux. Liquids can cause food to expand in your body, and they increase the volume of foods inside of your body. Instead, consider eating your meals first, and then enjoy your beverage about fifteen minutes after your meal is through.

178.   Try wearing loose clothes if you have acid reflux. Do what you can to avoid having anything that fits tightly near your middle area. This can cause unnecessary pressure on the stomach and worsen your acid reflux symptoms. You may resume wearing tight clothes after your symptoms are dealt with. In the mean time, try sticking with comfortable and stretchy clothes.

179.   If you smoke, you need to quit. Obviously, there are many reasons why you should quit, but if you suffer from acid reflux, this is yet another reason. Smoking slows down your digestion and reduces your saliva production, which worsens acid reflux symptoms. In addition, smoking harms your LES muscle, further worsening your acid reflux. Quitting this terrible habit can significantly improve your acid reflux, not to mention all the other benefits.

180.   Try to limit food consumption in the hours leading up to bed. Once you are in a resting state, your body is not able to digest food efficiently. When you eat close to bedtime, you will probably be awoken from heartburn.

181.   Make exercise a part of your healthy eating plan. Moderate exercise can facilitate the process involved in digesting your food properly, and it can also help you to lose excess pounds. Both of these things can have a positive effect on acid reflux problems. Make a point to work out at a moderate level at least three times a week for best results.

182.   Reduce the amount of caffeine that you consume during the day to help with your acid reflux. Caffeine can cause gas to build up in your stomach, which can lead to inflammation. Try not to drink a lot of coffee or soda during the day to limit the extremity of your condition.

183.   Eating smaller, more frequent meals is great for acid reflux sufferers. The first thing this change does is boosts your metabolism. The second benefit is that your stomach won't become huge like when you eat a larger meal, so less pressure will be placed on it, ensuring food and acid don't pass back up your esophagus.

184.   Shedding the pounds is a great way to control acid reflux. The heavier you are, the more weight is put on your abdomen, pushing the contents of your stomach upward. Also, increased body fat seems to exude chemicals into the system which causes digestion to slow to a crawl and even malfunction.

185.   Avoid constricting clothes if you suffer from heartburn. You can suffer heartburn problems wearing clothes that fit too tight. These clothes can put pressure on your abdominal area and stomach, pushing acids up to your throat, leading to uncomfortable heartburn. Your clothes should be comfortable and loose, and avoid tightening your belt excessively.

186.   Enjoy your food. If you savor each bite, investigating the flavors and truly allowing yourself to taste it, you will chew more and even eat less. Your stomach will realize it's full when you eat slowly, which allows you to keep your weight in check by eating less and also keep your stomach from overfilling.

187.   It is important to avoid vigorous exercise if you deal with GERD. When you are compressing the stomach violently, you'll find that acid makes its way up into your esophagus.

Instead, engage in moderate activity which helps you lose weight, stay in shape and yet ensures that acid stays where it belongs.

188.   There are some foods which people who suffer from acid reflux must avoid. These include high-fat foods, alcohol, drinks with caffeine, anything with mint in it, chocolate, citrus, anything with tomato in it, foods with spices in them, peppers, garlic, carbonated drinks and onions. You may find your acid reflux flares with many other foods as well, so make a list.

189.   It is a good idea to raise the head of your bed if you have been experiencing acid reflux issues frequently. When you are lying flat, it gives the stomach contents an easier way of refluxing. You should raise the mattress about 6-8 inches in order to get the best results.

190.   Many people like to lie down and relax after eating a big meal. This is bad for the digestive system and can lead to acid reflux. Instead, try walking around or standing to give the food a chance to digest. Wat at least two hours after eating to lie down. Also, elevate your body while sleeping.

191.   It may not be wise to exercise immediately after eating. Food that is in your stomach can be forced up into your esophagus when your lower abdominal muscles contract while exercising. Wait for a couple of hours before you work out.

192.   Don't just treat the symptoms of acid reflux with antacids. This does nothing to help reverse the damage caused to the esophagus caused by acid. You'll need to make lifestyle changes that prevent acid reflux from occurring to allow the esophagus to heal itself and prevent serious problems in the future.

193.   There are certain foods that trigger acid reflux. Therefore, it's in your best interest to avoid these if possible. One example is chocolate. While dark chocolate doesn't appear to be as bad as high-fat milk chocolate, they both contain caffeine and cocoa, which are both known to cause acid reflux.

194.   The food you consume each day will make a difference in your reflux. Avoiding acidic foods, peppers, greasy foods and alcoholic beverages could help. These foods and drinks could be causing the problem. Also, avoid eating less than three hours before you bed time. Going to bed

with a full stomach could make for a rough night and morning.

195.   Exercise daily to help reduce acid reflux. These exercises should be low impact exercises such as walking. Gravity is known to help decrease the odds of acid reflux; therefore, go for a walk after eating to lessen the effects of stomach upset and increased stomach acids. Exercising will also help you lose weight which will aid in reducing acid reflux.

196.   If over the counter medicine isn't giving you acid reflux relief, try pineapple for a more natural solution. Pineapple contains bromelain, which has been shown to lessen acid reflux symptoms. Bromelain is only present in fresh pineapple or fresh pineapple juice, however. Canned pineapple and store bought juices will not contain bromelain.

197.   For children who have acid reflux disease, the only thing that may work for them is time. When a person is younger, their digestive systems have not yet matured. This makes it easier for acid to produce, thus, increase acid reflux symptoms. Once they get older, the problem should go away.

198.   Give slippery elm lozenges a try. Slippery elm bark, the main ingredient in these natural lozenges, coats your digestive tract in a protective layer. When it is in lozenges, it relieves the coughing that comes with acid reflux and it soothes throat irritation. These lozenges are found in many health food stores.

199.   Learn stress coping techniques. Being stressed out can cause you to tense up your body and this causes you to contract some, or all, of your stomach muscles, causing acid reflux symptoms. Learn how to better handle stressful situations and you'll find out you may have much less stomach troubles.

200.   It is best for people with acid reflux to avoid certain beverages. Drinks like soda, energy drinks and coffee are all big causes of acid reflux. The caffeine content is usually the culprit and can cause the stomach to produce large amounts of stomach acid. They can also irritate the lining of the stomach.

201.   Tight clothes could make your digestion harder. If you often suffer from acid reflux, try wearing pants that are more comfortable. Do not hesitate to purchase pants that fit more loosely or wear softer fabrics than denim. You should

also avoid wearing belts that could put pressure on your stomach.

202.   Look for dairy products that are naturally low in fat, and you can relieve some of the acid reflux symptoms you may have been experiencing. Dairy that is high and fat can negatively affect the stomach and create a huge problem for people that suffer from acid reflux. You will have to work on getting used to the change in flavor.

203.   Slow down! When you eat more slowly, your body is able to keep up with what is being deposited in your stomach. This means that it will know that it is full when it truly is full, and you will eat less. If you overeat, you'll find your acid reflux goes crazy.

204.   Don't just assume your acid reflux is a fact of life or consequence of your active lifestyle. If you find yourself suffering through frequent bouts of discomfort related to acid reflux, see your doctor. It may be something you ate or an indication that you need to slow down in life, but it could also be something else you need to take care of.

205.   When you are at a healthy weight, it is less likely that you will suffer from GERD. This

condition occurs when fat weighs down on the stomach. Losing weight and getting trim can help keep your stomach acid in your stomach, where it belongs.

206.   Fatty food should be avoided. The chemicals released from breaking down all that fat will cause your esophageal sphincter to relax. In addition, these type of foods make you prone for weight gain. People who are overweight struggle even more with acid reflux. Eat healthy and stay healthy!

207.   Limit your liquid intake with meals if you're prone to acid reflux. Even healthy beverages like water can fill up your stomach fast, creating conditions that are conducive to acid reflux. Sip your beverage conservatively and never gulp it down. Wait a half an hour after a big meal to enjoy quenching your thirst.

208.   Never, ever, EVER lie down after you eat! Even if you have only had a few bites, you may find that food comes back to haunt you in short order if you lie down. Eat all meals at least two hours before lying down for a nap or overnight to ensure that acid doesn't sneak back up your esophagus.

209.   If you suffer with acid reflux, understand how gravity can work in your favor. Sitting upright will help keep food and fluids down after meals, so keep yourself straight. Avoid lying down or even slightly reclining in your favorite chair as this will exacerbate reflux symptoms quickly. Try going for a short and healthy walk instead!

210.   The food you consume each day will make a difference in your reflux. Avoiding acidic foods, peppers, greasy foods and alcoholic beverages could help. These foods and drinks could be causing the problem. Also, avoid eating less than three hours before you bed time. Going to bed with a full stomach could make for a rough night and morning.

211.   You should never lay down after a meal. The digestive tract can have trouble while you are laying down. Remaining upright can avoid issues with your acid reflux and keep you feeling healthy.

212.   Try to drink mostly in between meals if you suffer from acid reflux. A full stomach puts pressure on your esophageal sphincter. When you esophageal sphincter is compressed, your

food and stomach acid can go into your esophagus.

213.	Losing some weight can help with your acid reflux. Being overweight can contribute to heartburn. The extra pounds can cause excess pressure on the stomach making the LES or lower esophageal sphincter relax causing backflow. Extra body fat can also release some chemicals that interfere with normal digestion. Losing a few pounds can relieve many of these symptoms and keep heartburn to a minimum.

214.	Exercise regularly but moderately. Your acid reflux problem should not be as bad if you are in shape and live an active lifestyle. Avoid exercising intensely or your stomach could become upset. You could for instance go for walks everyday or find a new hobby that allows you to be more active.

215.	If excess pounds are plaguing you, work to lose them. Extra weight, particularly around the middle, can negatively affect acid reflux. It could cause stomach acid to rise up into the esophagus. This can end up causing an erosion of your esophageal lining. Staying healthy and exercising will help immensely.

216. What are your trigger foods? There are some foods that are known to trigger acid reflux. Some examples of these foods are spicy, fried or fatty, citrus fruits, caffeine, alcohol, mints or items that have mint flavoring, tomatoes, onions, garlic and carbonated beverages. Triggers vary from person to person, so continue to enjoy items that don't cause you problems.

217. Avoid lying down after you eat for at least two hours. Instead, get up and walk around to help your digestive tract work properly. The first two hours after eating is the perfect time to do the dishes, clean the house and go for a walk. Additionally, if your acid reflux flares up while you sleep, use risers to slightly elevate the head of your bed to help avoid stomach acids from going into your esophagus.

218. Boost the head of your bed. This tilts your head upwards and ensures your esophagus is never on the same parallel as your stomach. Imagine lying a full glass of water down on a table - the contents will pour out. The same happens to your stomach when you lay flat.

219. If you are not too keen on the idea of taking medication to control your acid reflux, there is still something you can do to. Many foods can

naturally help you combat your acid reflux. Herbal licorice has the ability to naturally coat your stomach with a protective gel when it is taken in tincture or tea form.

220.   Chew your food. The more you chew your food, the less work your stomach will have to do. This also slows down the rate at which you are eating, which allows your stomach to keep up with its fullness level. Once you've eaten enough, your stomach will alert your brain and you'll feel full.

221.   You may need to change your diet if you suffer from acid reflux disease. Sugary and processed foods increase the amount of acid that is produced in your stomach, the cause of acid reflux disease. Fruits and vegetables are great foods to eat that do not cause or worsen acid reflux.

222.   If you suffer with acid reflux, understand how gravity can work in your favor. Sitting upright will help keep food and fluids down after meals, so keep yourself straight. Avoid lying down or even slightly reclining in your favorite chair as this will exacerbate reflux symptoms quickly. Try going for a short and healthy walk instead!

223.   To thicken the mucuous lining of the stomach, try slippery elm. As a result, the lining of your stomach is protected. A tablespoon or two mixed with a cup of water before bed will often provide some relief.

224.   Many people like to lie down and relax after eating a big meal. This is bad for the digestive system and can lead to acid reflux. Instead, try walking around or standing to give the food a chance to digest. Wat at least two hours after eating to lie down. Also, elevate your body while sleeping.

225.   Learn your trigger foods. When you know what foods or beverages cause you acid reflux, you can avoid them to keep your symptoms to a minimum. Some foods that often cause symptoms are foods that are fried, fatty, spicy and carbonated drinks. These are just some examples and what bothers someone else, might not bother you.

226.   You should limit your alcohol consumption. Alcohol consumption is a major cause of excessive production of stomach acids. If you would like a drink, limit yourself to one or two servings of an alcoholic drink to does not cause symptoms of acid reflux.

227.   See a doctor. Many people think that acid reflux is something that can be treated at home. While this is true to some extent, you may be missing out on valuable insight and effective treatment. There are many causes of acid reflux, and your doctor can help you identify the root of the problem and devise a treatment plan tailored to your needs.

228.   Speak to a doctor if you feel like your acid reflux is not improving from the antacids that you are taking on a daily basis. Sometimes, you may need a serious form of medication that you doctor can prescribe, which can improve your symptoms. A professional's diagnosis may be the solution to your acid reflux issues.

229.   Chew gum after your meals. Believe it or not, chewing gum can help alleviate acid reflux because it encourages saliva production. Saliva helps eliminate stomach acid. In addition, you will likely swallow more often, which further helps clear acid. Aim to chew cinnamon or fruit-flavored gum rather than mint because mint could worsen your acid reflux.

230.   Avoid lying down after you eat for at least two hours. Instead, get up and walk around to

help your digestive tract work properly. The first two hours after eating is the perfect time to do the dishes, clean the house and go for a walk. Additionally, if your acid reflux flares up while you sleep, use risers to slightly elevate the head of your bed to help avoid stomach acids from going into your esophagus.

231.   If you are big into exercising, be moderate about your high-impact exercises. Major exertion in these hardcore fitness regimens can actually make your acid reflux worse. Instead, mix it up and get some time with more moderate fitness routines. A great choice is a long walk at a medium speed.

232.   Are you suffering with the painful heartburn associated with acid reflux? A natural solution to alleviate this pain can be found in your kitchen. Juicing can help give you relief. Cabbage juice, carrot juice and aloe vera juice are nutrient sources that provide relief. Since these juices sooth the esophagus, they can bring you safe relief.

233.   Avoid lying down after having some food. You need to wait between two and three hours before lying down, and even more after a large meal. If possible, go for a short walk to get some

exercise and sit until the digestion process is over. It is best to have your diner several hours before going to bed.

234.	Make sure that you chew all of your food very thoroughly before you swallow it. The more you chew it, the easier it will be for the food to mix with digestive enzymes. As a good point of reference, you should chew every bite of food 10 times before you swallow it.

235.	Do you often drink coffee? This beverage could upset your stomach enough to cause painful acid reflux. If you usually have coffee for your breakfast, get rid of this habit and find another beverage to start your day. Have coffee only in small quantities and avoid strong coffee as much as possible.

236.	If you are suffering from acid reflux several times a week and cannot find relief, you should visit your physician. You doctor may be able to prescribe medicines to limit the effects of acid reflux. Additionally, acid reflux can be a sign of a more serious problem such as esophageal cancer.

237.	If you have acid reflux disease, you may want to consider using Proton Pump Inhibitors, or PPIs. This is a medication is prescribed your doctor and is used to stop stomach acid from getting into your intestines and stomach. Obviously, if there is no acid in your stomach, it cannot come up through the esophagus either.

238.   You may need to balance out hydrochloric acid amounts in your body if you want to reduce acid reflux and its symptoms. You can do this, for instance, by using sea salt rather than table salt. Sea salt has chloride and minerals that are good for the stomach and prevent acid.

239.   Try drinking in between meals instead of during them. This will help you manage hunger, as it is likely that you are more thirsty than you are hungry. Acid will stay out of your esophagus more often if you do most of your beverage drinking outside of your meal time frames.

240.   We truly are what we eat. If we eat high-fat foods, we will become obese and be at risk for acid reflux. It is important that we instead focus on low-acid foods, which are lean and healthy. Choose vegetables and whole-grain carbohydrates along with lean protein for your meals to curb your suffering.

241.   If you plan to exercise rigorously, drink lots of water while you work out. This not only hydrates you; it helps to aid in digestion. It also

washes acid down and out of your esophagus, keeping it in your stomach where it belongs. If this still doesn't help, talk to your doctor about medications.

242.   Cinnamon gum is a good dessert to get accustomed to. Your salivary glands make more saliva when you chew. The benefit of saliva is that the stomach's acid can be neutralized. Since you swallow more when you chew gum, this will also wash down any acid remaining in your throat. You may find fruit flavored gum gives you the same effect. Mint flavored gum causes the esophageal sphincter to relax, adding to the problem.

243.   In order to ameliorate the pain and discomfort of acid reflux, consider breaking your daily food intake into five or so smaller meals instead of three main ones. This helps prevent you from overloading your digestive system at any one time, making acids work more effectively in smaller amounts. You will soon start to notice a real change in your symptoms for the better.

244.   Wait to exercise after you eat. If you put off your exercise by at least an hour, the food will have a better chance to digest. Physical exertion

right after you eat could cause the food to move back up toward the esophagus. This could be very uncomfortable and hard to fight.

245.   To reduce the risk of acid reflux, lose those extra pounds. Obesity often occurs with acid reflux. Just losing a small amount of weight can help. Adopt a healthy diet that includes reasonable quantities of many different foods instead of going on a crash diet.

246.   Try to eat slowly. Stop eating before you feel stuffed. Be sure to sit at the table and eat slowly, chew carefully and savor your food. When you eat too fast or continue eating when you feel stuffed, your symptoms will become worse. You can slow everything down by laying down your fork after each bite.

247.   If you are a pregnant, there is a chance that the weight of the baby is pushing against your stomach and causing your acid reflux to form. Speak to your doctor concerning the best actions to take during your pregnancy.

248.   A lozenge containing slippery elm may give you some relief. The main ingredient, slippery elm bark, will coat your digestive system with a protective layer. This type of lozenge soothes the

throat and relieves hoarseness and coughing that often accompany acid reflux. You can find them at any health food stores and natural food stores near you.

249.   Immediately after you have consumed a meal, do not lie flat. This can cause the food you have eaten to remain trapped in your esophagus, worsening acid reflux. Instead, walk around and remain upright for at least two hours. Doing this will assist in digestion, which will relieve your acid reflux.

250.   Tell your doctor about all of the medications that you are taking at the moment, as there can be a relation between them and your acid reflux. Medications can worsen your symptoms and reduce the effectiveness of your stomach and esophageal function. A drug-free lifestyle may be the answer to your acid reflux.

251.   Enjoy a stick of gum after your meals. The chewing motions helps increase your digestive juices which helps your body process its food faster. Additionally, avoid chewing minty type gum, such as peppermint or spearmint, as these are known to relax stomach muscles. Instead, opt for either cinnamon or fruit flavored gum.

252.   Increasing your vitamin D exposure can be a great way to help reduce your acid reflux. Vitamin D can be naturally found outside in the sun's rays. Getting enough of it is important to ensure that your body is producing enough antimicrobial peptides that can help eliminate infections in the esophagus.

253.   Do not stuff yourself with food. The amount of food you eat in one sitting has a big impact on your acid reflux symptoms. Instead of eating until you are uncomfortable, eat until you feel satisfied. This allows your stomach do properly do its job and can cut down on irritating symptoms.

254.   Stay away from acidic foods. They can both cause and exacerbate acid reflux. While this is by no means a comprehensive list, try to avoid oranges, tomatoes, grapefruit and vinegar. If you can't cut them out of your diet completely, at least try to avoid eating them in the evenings, so acid reflux doesn't strike when it is time for bed.

255.   Chew your food. The more you chew your food, the less work your stomach will have to do. This also slows down the rate at which you are eating, which allows your stomach to keep up with its fullness level. Once you've eaten enough,

your stomach will alert your brain and you'll feel full.

256.   Make sure you eat dinner at least three hours before bed. When you are in an upright position, the food and stomach acid gets pulled down into your stomach. If you lie down, your stomach acids can rise into your esophagus. Thus, you need to delay going to bed.

257.   If you suffer from acid reflux symptoms at night time, you may need to change the way you sleep. You should be laying on your back, with the upper half of your body propped up by a few pillows. When you lay flat, whether on your back, stomach or side, you are allowing acid to come up through the esophagus.

258.   Always keep gravity in mind. Remember that acid is being held down, so when you position your body in a way where down isn't towards your feet, problems will ensue. Keep your head up and your stomach uncompressed, then you should be able to find relief from acid reflux all day long.

259.   Stop smoking if you are trying to rid yourself of issues with acid reflux. Many people do not know this, but smoking causes the muscles in the

esophagus to relax. This can create some of the symptoms associated with acid reflux, so quit if you are trying to make things better.

260.   If you are pregnant and experiencing acid reflux, try to relax. This problem is often no longer an issue after you have the baby. It is a symptom of the baby pushing on all of your innards causing the acid in your belly to rise. Watch what you eat and avoid laying down until an hour has passed after you eat.

261.   If you have acid reflux symptoms during the day and at night, gum might solve the problem. Chewing gum helps you produce more saliva. Saliva is a natural neutralizer of stomach acid. If you can, try chewing gum even through the night to try to decrease your level of discomfort through the night and into the morning.

262.   Stay away from alcohol if you need to get rid of acid reflux. Alcohol has many bad effects on your health. Among them are damage to the lining of the stomach and an increase in stomach acids. Keep your alcohol intake to a minimum, or none at all, to avoid the symptoms of acid reflux.

263.   Drinking a large amount of liquid while eating can lead to acid reflux. You may not think about it, but liquids also add to the volume of food in your stomach. When the volume of food is too great, it overpowers your body's resources to keep food in your stomach. Limit the amount of liquid you drink while eating, or only drink between meals.

264.   If you are overweight or obese and you have acid reflux disease, you should do your best to lose weight. When you are overweight, organs surrounding the stomach could actually push into the stomach, causing too much acid to form. It could even weaken your esophagus, making it more likely for acid to come up.

265.   You need to relax. Don't eat when you're upset or you will increase your acid build-up. When your meal is finished, relax by doing some deep breathing or meditation. Avoid lying down right after eating.

266.   If you have constant acid reflux, you need to do moderate exercise on a regular basis. Going for a walk or doing some water aerobics are excellent ways to help address symptoms. Your body is in an upright position and gravity will

help aid digestion and keep your food in your stomach where it belongs.

267.   Do not drink at mealtime if you want to lower the risk of reflux. Drinking at mealtime increases your stomach volume. When this happens, pressure is applied to your lower esophageal sphincter, raising the risk of experiencing reflux. Have a drink in between meals as opposed to while you are eating; this will help to reduce the risk.

268.   Keep excess fats out of your diet. When you eat foods that are really high in fats, you are setting yourself up to have more problems with your acid reflux. Those fats make it tough for your body to empty the stomach properly which then leads to increased reflux issues. Stick to leaner foods.

269.   Keep your clothing loose and comfortable. Tight clothing can put extra pressure on the abdominal region, bringing about problems like GERD and reflux. Never try to push yourself into a pair of jeans or wear a girdle if you suffer from such problems. Staying comfortable is key if you want to avoid reflux discomfort.

270.   If you find you are having trouble swallowing, see a doctor as soon as possible. Acid reflux can damage the esophagus, leading to scarring of the area. This scarring then leads to inflammation and your esophagus can literally close. This is when medical intervention is a must to ensure you remain healthy.

271.   If you're experiencing acid reflux lately, try a new diet that consists of low-acid foods. Avoid spicy or acidic foods and eat your food slowly. If you still get acid reflux, it's probably time to check in with your doctor. Although your problem may not be serious, it may require medication that your doctor can recommend or prescribe.

272.   There are some foods which people who suffer from acid reflux must avoid. These include high-fat foods, alcohol, drinks with caffeine, anything with mint in it, chocolate, citrus, anything with tomato in it, foods with spices in them, peppers, garlic, carbonated drinks and onions. You may find your acid reflux flares with many other foods as well, so make a list.

273.   Pregnancy often causes acid reflux. The baby's growth tends to crowd the contents of the stomach, forcing acid into the esophagus. Eating non-acidic foods that are low in fat will help

prevent reflux. You can also try soothing teas which help to neutralize the acids in your stomach.

274.   When you want to reach for a natural treatment for heartburn, consider licorice. You need to choose DGL licorice which doesn't contain glycyrrhizic acid and therefore will not cause hypertension. Chewable tablets are your best bet before meals, and they can be found affordably at natural food retailers and health supplement shops.

275.   Exercising after eating can be a disaster if you're suffering from acid reflux. Your food can be pushed up into the esophagus as your abdominal muscles are flexing. Wait a few hours before you engage in any physical activity.

276.   You want to avoid foods that contain a high amount of acid in order to reduce acid reflux attacks. Examples of foods that are known to have a high acidic content are grapefruit, tomatoes, and pineapple. If you do have a history of issues after eating these foods, it may be best to avoid eating them late at night, or entirely.

277.   Do not drink alcohol if you want to live free of acid reflux. Besides causing acid to begin to

build up and eat away at your stomach lining, alcohol worsens acid reflux. Do not drink too much while out with friends if you don't want a lot of discomfort later that night.

278.   Stop smoking. Smoking can cause the muscles that control the esophageal sphincter between the stomach and esophagus to relax. When this happens, stomach acid can escape from the stomach and into your esophagus, causing that familiar burning sensation. If you are a smoker and frequently get bouts of heartburn, it may be time to quit or at least reduce your habit.

279.   Chew a stick of gum if you feel like your acid reflux issue is not under control at night. A stick of gum can increase the amount of saliva that you have in your mouth, which can help push down the acid that is getting into your esophagus from your stomach.

280.   Losing some weight can help with your acid reflux. Being overweight can contribute to heartburn. The extra pounds can cause excess pressure on the stomach making the LES or lower esophageal sphincter relax causing backflow. Extra body fat can also release some chemicals that interfere with normal digestion.

Losing a few pounds can relieve many of these symptoms and keep heartburn to a minimum.

281.   Try a spoonful of honey. While there is no hard evidence that honey treats acid reflux, it is very useful to soothe and relieve the painful burning associated with it. Honey will coat your esophagus in a protective and soothing layer, and help neutralize some of the acid. If you are looking for some relief until you can identify and treat the cause of your heartburn, a little honey can be just what you need to get back to sleep.

282.   Try to eat slowly. Eating too fast will cause acid reflux to strike. If you find that you have trouble with this, make an effort to take a bite and then put your utensil down. This will ensure that you don't put too much food in your mouth at any given time.

283.   Chew some mint-free gum after every meal. Chewing gum helps with producing saliva, which can neutralize stomach acid. It also causes frequent swallowing, which can clear aggravating acid away from the esophagus quicker. Mint flavored gums can relax the LES and worsen a reflux, so try going with fruit or cinnamon gums.

284.   Quit smoking immediately to prevent acid reflux from occurring. Smoking cigarettes can increase the nicotine content that enters your body, which can damage your esophagus. A damaged esophagus can lead to more acid buildup in your body and trigger acid reflux episodes. Also, smoking will help you to live a healthier lifestyle and reduce esophageal cancer.

285.   It is best for people with acid reflux to avoid certain beverages. Drinks like soda, energy drinks and coffee are all big causes of acid reflux. The caffeine content is usually the culprit and can cause the stomach to produce large amounts of stomach acid. They can also irritate the lining of the stomach.

286.   When you have acid reflux disease it can be difficult to eat foods that are acidic such as tomato sauce and salsa. If you have been steering clear of these foods out of fear of discomfort, you no longer have to avoid them altogether. Taking an antacid prior to eating these types of foods can help you avoid experiencing acid reflux.

287.   The most significant factor attributed with acid reflux is being overweight. Those who are obese are two times more likely to have GERD than someone who is at a healthy weight. The

pressure on your stomach of all the extra pounds can cause the esophageal sphincter to relax, allowing acid to give you trouble.

288.   If you suffer from acid reflux symptoms at night time, you may need to change the way you sleep. You should be laying on your back, with the upper half of your body propped up by a few pillows. When you lay flat, whether on your back, stomach or side, you are allowing acid to come up through the esophagus.

289.   For a good night's sleep, consider putting a wedge under your mattress to raise your head up to keep acid where it belongs. You can be creative about what you use. Boards, old books, bricks and so forth will all work just as well to elevate the head of your bed. There are beds which are electronically controlled which you can use as well.

290.   While vinegar tastes great on salads or french fries, anyone with acid reflux should avoid eating it. Vinegar, along with citrus fruit and tomatoes, is high in acid, and the more acid you eat, the more acid will return up your esophagus and cause you pain and discomfort after meals.

291.   Don't confuse acid reflux with GERD! The latter can be a very serious indication that you've got other problems, whereas most often acid reflux is related to eating and lifestyle. If you're not sure, see your doctor right away and find out what's going on with your digestive system right away.

292.   Do not take large bites when you are eating a meal if you want to feel comfortable and prevent the burning sensation from acid reflux. It is important for your body to break down the food that you put in your mouth, especially meats. Take small bites and chew your food for at least 10 seconds to feel comfortable during and after your meal.

293.   Lose weight by going to the gym and performing cardiovascular exercises if you want to limit your acid reflux symptoms. If you are overweight, you will have a better chance of acid reflux building in your stomach and causing heartburn. Exercising can help with your heartburn and improve your health at the same time.

294.   If you have acid reflux, you should engage in moderate exercise. Going for a walk or doing some water aerobics are excellent ways to help

address symptoms. The body will be upright, causing gravity to aid in digestion.

295.   Try to create separation between your workout regimen and the meals that you eat during the day. It is important to give your body this rest so that it can rehabilitate from your intense session of working out. This time will give your stomach the opportunity to become strong so that it can break down your food efficiently.

296.   Slowly consume your meals to alleviate your acid reflux. Make sure you actually enjoy your food. Don't stuff yourself. Stop eating before you become too full.

297.   Try bending your knees back and forth for at least 10 minutes during the day and night. This motion can help improve the flow of liquids down your esophagus and help facilitate your acid reflux symptoms. You can do this in the comfort of your own home or as part of your exercise regimen for relief.

298.   Increasing your vitamin D exposure can be a great way to help reduce your acid reflux. Vitamin D can be naturally found outside in the sun's rays. Getting enough of it is important to

ensure that your body is producing enough antimicrobial peptides that can help eliminate infections in the esophagus.

299.   Add a few fermented foods to your regular diet if you are trying to eliminate any acid reflux issues you have. These foods help to stabilize the stomach if you eat them in moderate amounts. Foods that are including in this category include all types of pickles, kimchee and sauerkraut.

300.   Look for your acid reflux trigger foods. Every body is different, and there will be certain types of foods that really kick your acid reflux into high gear. Keep note of times when that occurs and analyze what you ate. If you see recurring patterns, look to strategically change your diet.

301.   Try following a gluten-free diet. Gluten is a protein that is found in wheat, barley, and rye. For some people, gluten can actually cause acid reflux. If your acid reflux is severe, you could even have a life-threatening condition called celiac disease. This is a condition where your acid reflux is so bad that it is literally eating away your insides. Have yourself tested for this condition if you have extreme acid reflux, and if you do, you

can eliminate your acid reflux by going gluten free.

302.   If you are constantly stressed out, you need to find a way to reduce your stress. Stress does not cause acid reflux itself, but, when you are stressed, you tend to get involved in bad habits, like drinking, eating too much and smoking. These activities make acid reflux worse. Thus, lower your stress, and you can limit your acid reflux problems.

303.   Get plenty of exercise and lose weight. Carrying excess pounds can cause acid reflux, as it puts more pressure on the abdominal. This pushes acids up into the esophagus. Even losing a few pounds can help. Statistics indicate that about 35% of overweight people suffer from heartburn or acid reflux.

304.   If you're suffering from acid reflux while sleeping, try putting a wedge below your mattress. It raises up your head, keeping symptoms from increasing. Anything that angles the bed up will work, including some books or wooden blocks. If you can afford it, you could invest in an electronic bed that you can adjust with the push of a button.

305.   It is time for you to quit smoking. Smoking exacerbates acid reflux and actually can be a cause of it. Smoking slows down digestion and saliva production, both of which worsen reflux. It also weakens the muscles of the esophageal sphincter as well. So stop smoking now.

306.   If you suffer with acid reflux, understand how gravity can work in your favor. Sitting upright will help keep food and fluids down after meals, so keep yourself straight. Avoid lying down or even slightly reclining in your favorite chair as this will exacerbate reflux symptoms quickly. Try going for a short and healthy walk instead!

307.   Avoid consuming spicy foods like peppers and hot sauces. These food items work to heighten the acids that build up inside the digestive system, causing your condition to be worsened. Kicking spicy foods out of your diet can often promote instant relief.

308.   Avoid eating spicy foods including those with hot peppers in them. These foods can lead to painful acid reflux after eating, so not eating them can easily remedy your discomfort. Instead, focus on spices which don't lead to pain, such as

cinnamon or herbs. They taste great and leave you comfortable post-meal.

309.   Wait to exercise after you eat. If you put off your exercise by at least an hour, the food will have a better chance to digest. Physical exertion right after you eat could cause the food to move back up toward the esophagus. This could be very uncomfortable and hard to fight.

310.   The food you consume each day will make a difference in your reflux. Avoiding acidic foods, peppers, greasy foods and alcoholic beverages could help. These foods and drinks could be causing the problem. Also, avoid eating less than three hours before you bed time. Going to bed with a full stomach could make for a rough night and morning.

311.   You want to avoid foods that contain a high amount of acid in order to reduce acid reflux attacks. Examples of foods that are known to have a high acidic content are grapefruit, tomatoes, and pineapple. If you do have a history of issues after eating these foods, it may be best to avoid eating them late at night, or entirely.

312.   A moderate exercise plan that includes activities like walking that keeps you standing up

is best for acid reflux sufferers. Walking, for example, can help improve symptoms in several ways. For example, the upright position facilitates digestion. Also, it can facilitate weight loss, which also improves acid reflux symptoms. Light to moderate exercise helps acid reflux. Extreme exercise can make it worse.

313.   Exercise regularly but moderately. Your acid reflux problem should not be as bad if you are in shape and live an active lifestyle. Avoid exercising intensely or your stomach could become upset. You could for instance go for walks everyday or find a new hobby that allows you to be more active.

314.   What you drink could play a major role in whether you have acid reflux symptoms or not. Carbonated beverages, such as soda, increase stomach acid production, thus, increasing acid that comes up through the esophagus. Caffeinated beverages also have the same effect. Try to stay away from these drinks and stick to water.

315.   Try bending your knees back and forth for at least 10 minutes during the day and night. This motion can help improve the flow of liquids down your esophagus and help facilitate your

acid reflux symptoms. You can do this in the comfort of your own home or as part of your exercise regimen for relief.

316.   Consider keeping a food diary if you suffer from reflux. There are several foods that are often found to be acid reflux triggers for some individuals. They include things like tomatoes, onions, coffee, tea and even chocolate. If you keep a food diary, you can easily spot when your reflux problems are taking place and which foods appear to be causing the problems.

317.   There are many different symptoms that can accompany acid reflux, outside of the obvious burning in your esophagus after meals. Chest pain, pain after meals, a bitter taste in your mouth, a sore or hoarse throat or a cough are all indications that you might be suffering from acid reflux disease.

318.   Pregnant women often experience acid reflux, especially in the last trimester of their pregnancy. This is caused when the baby grows large enough to limit the amount of space in the abdomen of the mother. You can try wearing looser clothing, avoiding certain foods that seem to set it off, or ask your doctor which medication is safe for the baby.

319.   One thing you can do to help you get rid of your acid reflux is to eat your food slowly. This helps your digestive system catch up to you. Plus, you enjoy your food more this way as well. Eat smaller portions, and take your food in slowly like you actually want to enjoy your meal.

320.   After eating, avoid the urge to sit still or, worse yet, lie down. Food will settle and perhaps cause you to experience regurgitation, or acid coming up. Move around and sit upright so you food can digest properly.

321.   If you have acid reflux disease, you may want to consider using Proton Pump Inhibitors, or PPIs. This is a medication is prescribed your doctor and is used to stop stomach acid from getting into your intestines and stomach. Obviously, if there is no acid in your stomach, it cannot come up through the esophagus either.

322.   To sleep well at night and prevent acid reflux, you may want to place a wedge underneath the mattress in order to keep your head raised. A book, piece of wood or something else that is similarly shaped will also do the trick. Electronic beds which can raise the upper portion of the bed are also available too.

323. Skinny jeans are the enemy of the acid reflux sufferer! Wearing tight clothes can block up your digestive system, causing you a great deal of pain when acid begins to back up. Go for elastic waistbands until you have your acid reflux under control, then you can consider getting back into your tight fitting pants.

324. If you have been having any acid reflux symptoms over an extended period of time, make sure that you go in to be seen by a doctor. You may think that this condition is not that serious, but if it is not treated it can lead to more serious health issues, including ulcers and gastritis.

325. What you drink will affect your acid reflux just as much as what you eat. Anything with caffeine should be avoided. In addition, carbonated beverages will cause you to have issues, as will alcohol. Be mindful of what you consume, and try to stick with water whenever possible if you want to be on the safe side.

326. Do not take large bites when you are eating a meal if you want to feel comfortable and prevent the burning sensation from acid reflux. It is important for your body to break down the food that you put in your mouth, especially meats.

Take small bites and chew your food for at least 10 seconds to feel comfortable during and after your meal.

327.   Keep a journal of all of the foods that seem to be causing you to get acid reflux and the ones that are not. Steer clear of the foods that you see to be a problem in your life. Every person reacts differently to certain foods, so personalize your regimen to account for this.

328.   Try to drink mostly in between meals if you suffer from acid reflux. When your stomach is full of food an liquid, the lower esophageal sphincter is under constant pressure. This can cause it to allow the food and acid in your stomach to come back up into your esophagus and destroy the lining within.

329.   Try wearing loose clothes if you have acid reflux. Do what you can to avoid having anything that fits tightly near your middle area. This can cause unnecessary pressure on the stomach and worsen your acid reflux symptoms. You may resume wearing tight clothes after your symptoms are dealt with. In the mean time, try sticking with comfortable and stretchy clothes.

330.   A great way to eliminate your acid reflux is to switch your diet over to a plant based diet. Meat is a huge contributor to acid reflux. This seems to be contradictory because meats seem to be very alkaline when tested prior to consumption. The problem is that after meat is digested, it will leave a highly acidic residue within the body.

331.   Gluten is a potent acid reflux trigger food for many folks. Foods with gluten, such as oats, barely or wheat, need to be avoided by people who have acid reflux. A couple of grains that are helpful for digestion and contain the bodies' necessary fiber are quinoa and millet.

332.   Get medium-level exercise into your daily routine. Exercises such as walking for two miles can really help your digestion. As an added benefit, it can also help you lose weight which can again help your acid reflux issues. It's a win on both ways! Steer clear of high-level exercise though, as it can actually cause your acid reflux to spike.

333.   If you are big into exercising, be moderate about your high-impact exercises. Major exertion in these hardcore fitness regimens can actually make your acid reflux worse. Instead, mix it up

and get some time with more moderate fitness routines. A great choice is a long walk at a medium speed.

334.   Avoid constricting clothes if you suffer from heartburn. You can suffer heartburn problems wearing clothes that fit too tight. These clothes can put pressure on your abdominal area and stomach, pushing acids up to your throat, leading to uncomfortable heartburn. Your clothes should be comfortable and loose, and avoid tightening your belt excessively.

335.   Keep excess fats out of your diet. When you eat foods that are really high in fats, you are setting yourself up to have more problems with your acid reflux. Those fats make it tough for your body to empty the stomach properly which then leads to increased reflux issues. Stick to leaner foods.

336.   Look for your acid reflux trigger foods. Every body is different, and there will be certain types of foods that really kick your acid reflux into high gear. Keep note of times when that occurs and analyze what you ate. If you see recurring patterns, look to strategically change your diet.

337.   Exercising your abdominal muscles could cause acid reflux. You should get some exercise after eating to make digestion easier, but going for a walk is enough. Avoid lifting things or putting any kind of pressure on your abs. If your job requires you to be active immediately after your lunch break, choose your foods carefully.